Table of Contents

4.1. Summary of Key Points

4.2. Practical Tips for Maximizing Vitamin Absorption

Best Form of Vitamins for Absorption

1. Introduction to Vitamin Absorption

Vitamins are of two types - water-soluble and fat-soluble. The fat-soluble vitamins are vitamins A, D, E, and K, and the water-soluble vitamins are vitamin B and vitamin C. Among the two, fat-soluble vitamins are not absorbed in our body, and the rest are the vitamins that are directly absorbed into the bloodstream or digestive system by the body. There are two types of reserves in the body: active reserve and passive reserve. About 25% of the active reserve and 68% of the passive reserve of vitamin A is found in the liver. It was also observed that the storage capacity of the actively absorbed vitamin in the liver was 17-44 times higher than the absorption capacity of water-soluble vitamins. Non-storage of ascorbic acid (Vitamin C) in the body indicates the poor or no role of passive reserves. Fat-soluble Vitamins A, D, E, and K are the primary vitamins that have significant fat storage in our body except for vitamin D, which is stored in the inactive but is not the main fat storage one. Only vitamin A and vitamin E fat have significant fat storage. Moreover, the type of form in which vitamins are absorbed also plays an integral role in the processing and transportation in the body. In most cases, organic forms of absorption are preferred before inorganic, if any.

Vitamin absorption is the process by which the vitamins get absorbed and metabolized in your body. Vitamins are essential as they help prevent diseases, aid in keeping the skin and muscles healthy, help children grow, and are good for eyes. They have to be provided to the body through supplements or nutrition as they cannot be synthesized by the body. Hypovitaminosis can occur if there is an insufficient amount of vitamins absorbed and transported to the cells. Hypovitaminosis is a condition where the levels of one or more vitamins in the body are low.

1.1. Importance of Vitamin Absorption

There are 13 vitamins that the body absolutely needs: vitamins A, C, D, E, K, and eight B vitamins. For instance, vitamin A is necessary for vision, proper development, the immune system, and regular organ function; vitamin C aids in the protection of cells, helps the body absorb iron, and plays a significant role in the creation of connective tissue. Vitamin K aids in blood clotting, and E and D are necessary for immune function and bone health, respectively. These vitamins are essential to maintaining a stable life since they perform crucial functions in the body. However, the body is unable to generate the majority of them in adequate amounts, necessitating that they be consumed by diet or supplements. Many who ingest only a tiny portion of vitamins may obtain them using supplements, especially those who experience symptoms of a deficiency. Because of their water-soluble nature, B vitamins and vitamin C are not stored in the body like fat-soluble vitamins. To guarantee that we get enough of these nutrients, we need enough dietary sources or supplements daily. They will combine with binding proteins in the digestive tract and be absorbed like other dietary fats. Proper fat digestion, therefore, is required for efficient absorption.

Vitamins perform a myriad of crucial functions in the body, from regulating biochemical reactions to converting food into energy. It is critical that we're able to absorb our necessary vitamins effectively in order for the body to use them.

2. Factors Affecting Vitamin Absorption

It is important to understand that even the basic life-sustaining practice of food consumption can ultimately have a positive or negative effect on nutrient absorption. A diet that is highly processed, laden with excessive sugar and refined ingredients, and heavy in fat content may lead to reduced nutrient absorption overall, as well as poor overall health. On the other hand, incorporating a balanced diet filled with fruits, vegetables, whole grains, and lean protein sources can greatly enhance vitamin absorption in the body. A diet such as this would also contain many of the vitamins and minerals needed by the body for absorption and metabolism of other vitamins.

Today's grocery stores carry a huge variety of multivitamins and supplements, making it easier for people to maintain a more balanced diet and make sure their bodies are getting adequate nutrition. But as beneficial as these vitamin supplements may be, the body cannot make use of them without first successfully absorbing the various vitamins they contain. There are a number of factors that can contribute to enhanced vitamin absorption, or can work against it, and understanding this process can help one to ensure they're getting the vitamins and minerals they need from their supplements. In the sections that follow, absorption of specific vitamins will be covered in detail, but it is important to point out that the process involved in their absorption is very similar.

2.1. Bioavailability of Different Vitamin Forms

A high bioavailability vitamin, or vitamin with high bioavailability, can be defined as the extent to and rate of the absorption and subsequent utilization of a vitamin. Bioavailability is determined by evaluating the overall nature of the vitamin, and many factors can influence the extent and rate of vitamin absorption. Absorption is influenced by a compound's solubility. The solubility of a compound is a measure of the amount of that compound dissolvable in water. It is understood that all vitamins except A, D, E, and K are water-soluble. The low solubility of vitamins A, D, E, and K, coupled with their physiological states as fat-soluble vitamins, indicates a need for fats and other lipids in order to aid in their absorption. The structure of a compound is another important factor. The structure of compounds is of great importance when it comes to understanding their bioavailability. The different forms of a vitamin are defined based on the structure of a compound's functional group.

Every vitamin exists in different chemical compounds, which can greatly impact how a vitamin will be utilized by the body. The most bioavailable chemical form of a vitamin is referred to as its first-generation vitamin. These first-generation vitamins will generally have moderate to great bioavailability, with exceptions in a few fat-soluble vitamins. In contrast, the long-chain derivatives and synthetic analogs of these vitamins are the second and third generations of each vitamin. For the most part, these are minimally or poorly absorbed in the body.

3. Vitamin A

An essential nutrient, vitamin A is required for cell function and growth, as well as immune system performance. Vitamin A can be obtained through food and dietary supplements. The vitamin comes in three different categories, each with different addresses and impacts. Because retinol is readily absorbed and used by people, it's been shown to encourage vitamin A absorption better than beta-carotene. A variety of foods contain retinoids, such as meat and dairy items, including liver, milk, and cheese, to mention only a few. Beta-carotene, which is present in fruits and vegetables such as carrots, sweet potatoes, and spinach, is an important and healthful supply of carotenoid. Even if the body can use beta-carotene to produce vitamin A, some beta-carotene supplements can also be used as processed vitamin A for improved absorption. Always consult the nutrition label on the food item to ascertain the total vitamin A included in entire foods.

Vitamin A is a fat-soluble vitamin that is necessary for a healthy vision, a good immune function, and cell growth. It occurs naturally in the body in the forms of retinol and retinal, which are compounds known as preformed vitamin A. This type is a type of vitamin A that is readily absorbed and utilized for various biological processes. Found in meat, poultry, fish, and dairy foods, vitamin A is present in either organic compounds in which the carbon atoms are linked to each other, or inorganic compounds such as water and carbon dioxide. Moreover, beta-carotene is another form of vitamin A that may act as an antioxidant.

3.1. Retinol vs. Beta-Carotene

Retinol is found in animal foods such as eggs, milk, liver, and fish liver oil, and since it is ready-made vitamin A, it can be directly and easily absorbed into the body. Since the need for the body changes daily, as much as the body needs it, a balance sheet is of great importance. Different, especially in mail purchased omega-3 preformed vitamin A from fish oil from the fish state, cannot be found in the transit retinol are story vitamin D structures. In order to be absorbed into the body, it needs to be converted into retinol. The conversion of vitamin A from the beta-carotene found in plant foods varies according to the individual. If it is observed that the body needs a lot of vitamin A or if a large amount of retinol is needed on that day, preformed vitamin A can be preferred to meet the need in a shorter time. Preformed vitamin A (retinol) is often used in individuals with nutrient absorption problems and in case of need for short-term vitamin A replacement to reach sufficient levels. However, since it does not provide the same accidentally as beta-carotene, its long-term use can cause the accumulation of this vitamin in the body, whereas this risk is less in the use of beta-carotene.

Retinol vs. Beta-Carotene: Which one is best? The best way to consume vitamin A is in the form of beta-carotene (vitamin A precursor) and not retinol (preformed vitamin A) as beta-carotene usually converts into vitamin A according to the need of the body. Both beta-carotene (vitamin A precursor) and retinol (a pre-formed vitamin) are very good sources of vitamin A. Beta-carotene is a plant-sourced vitamin A precursor that our bodies convert to retinol. Retinol, on the other hand, is an active, pre-formed vitamin from animal sources. "Pre-formed" means it has already been converted into vitamin A and is ready for your body to use immediately. Both of these can be a great way to meet the body's needs for vitamin A, but each has its own unique features. Mostly, retinol is preferred over beta-carotene to meet the daily vitamin A needs, but sometimes, if there is a reason for that personalized need, beta-carotene can be preferred to meet the daily vitamin A need.

4. Vitamin B Complex

Unlike the water-soluble vitamins and minerals, which are absorbed by the small intestines, the B vitamins require a special mechanism for absorption due to their large size and high water solubility. Dietary cobalamin (B12) is bound to protein and is freed by food proteins in the stomach. Intrinsic factor (a protein produced by the stomach) is also needed for binding to and transporting vitamin B12. Absorption of B vitamins primarily occurs in the upper small intestine (the jejunum), which is the part of the small intestine fattened by many folds. Intestinal cells lining these folds and villi contain receptors that attach to circulating vitamin B, which is then transported into the body's blood supply. The B vitamins are widely distributed in animal and plant food products, so deficiency in any single B vitamin is rare and usually occurs as a result of inadequate intake or in association with malabsorption syndromes or other medical conditions. Each B vitamin is a distinct molecule and has a distinct receptor molecule on the intestines. This wide distribution of vitamin B with its large number of absorption sites and transport mechanisms represents an evolutionary adaptation of animal organisms to offering numerous opportunities for the absorption of a critical nutrient.

The B complex vitamins are actually a group of eight vitamins, which include thiamine (B1), riboflavin (B2), niacin (vitamin B3), pantothenic acid (B5), pyridoxine (B6), biotin (B7), folic acid (folate), and cobalamin (B12).

The B vitamins are important for normal energy production and the function of many cell types, tissues, and organs. These vitamins are involved in the metabolism of protein, fats, and carbohydrates and in animal and human nutrition are critical for supporting many cellular functions, including but not limited to: 1) brain health and the production of neurotransmitters, 2) the production of DNA/RNA, 3) fertility and pregnancy due to its role in methylation and cellular energy production, 4) the health of the nervous system, 5) and the maturation of red blood cells (which are needed to oxygenate the body and brain). As a family, the B vitamins are needed for regulation of the nervous system while some act as enzyme cofactors.

The essential nutrients your body needs: Benefits and offers to individuals with co-occurring disorders.

4.1. Different Forms of B Vitamins

Vitamins within the B group are not only chemically distinct; they also have varying properties inside the body and are used for different purposes. Currently, most of the B vitamins on the market for oral consumption will be present in a free form. Both the free form and activated co-enzymatic forms of B vitamins will each have properties and perform distinct biological functions. One of the more simplified examples is folic acid and the body's utilization of it. Some individuals might excrete a portion of free folic acid while the liver might take up the majority of activated methyl folate in circulation. So, between two doses of methyl folate, based on a person's methylation processes, some might have to take higher doses of methyl folate to even get lower plasma levels because their body, via liver, would be keeping and taking up the product of folic acid or methyl folate from circulation. In turn, free forms of folate and B vitamins, in general, have the potential to be excreted via urine as they cannot be taken up easily by the liver once the hepatic saturated level has been reached within the body. NAC, based on composition and methionine properties, can have a peptide bond which decreases B1 uptake too.

Vitamin B is actually made up of eight distinct vitamins, all of which are water-soluble. As a result, they cannot be stored in the body and need to be replenished daily. Of all the vitamins, B vitamins are perhaps the most complex. Each of the eight vitamins has a slightly different structure, something that impacts their functionality. There is also room for variation within the varieties of individual B vitamins due to slight differences in chemical structure. These differences relate to the composition of the various side chains. As a result, these differences can have an impact on how the body uses each individual vitamin.

5. Vitamin C

Absorption of Vitamin C, when ingested as Ester-C versus regular ascorbic acid, is a debated topic. A recent study published in the journal Antioxidants found that Ester-C has 217% greater absorption compared to ascorbic acid. In this study, 48 healthy subjects (30-74 years of age) consumed either 1000 mg of Ester-C or 1000 mg of ascorbic acid. Following consumption, blood was collected at baseline and 5 additional post-consumption time points. Fluorescence was evaluated using a MALDI-TOF/ME FC mass spectrophotometer. The Jellison formula was used to calculate the vitamin C transport rate from erythrocytes to plasma. The areas under the curve (AUC) measurements were taken over 6 hours. In the 48 participants, the AUC for vitamin C was 5887.3 µM/h for the Ester-C form, and 1853.6 µM/h for ascorbic acid, showing 217% greater absorption for Ester-C. In the 30-49, 50-59, 60-69 and over 70 age groups, the AUC was 5865.7, 9898.6, 5135.2 and 1116.0 µM/h for Ester-C. The AUC was 1975.8, 3381.1, and 803.1 µM/h for ascorbic acid; therefore, absorption with Ester-C was 197% more in the 30-49-year-olds, 192% in the 50-59-year-olds and 641% in the 60-69-year-olds and 139% more in the over 70-year-old age group.

Vitamin C is a potent antioxidant and has diverse physiological functions in the human body. Vitamin C is well known for its immune-supporting potential and its role in collagen formation. Regarding its absorption, a previous examination of Vitamin C products found huge differences between products in how much of this water-soluble vitamin is actually being delivered into the body. An article stated that regular ascorbic acid was less expensive and the better choice in an economic/efficacy balance. However, the Ester-C form was better for absorption but more expensive. Ester-C is a proprietary form of Vitamin C. Ester-C is made from the calcium salt of L-ascorbic acid. According to the Ester-C-specific trademark, when this ascorbate binds to a metabolite from the vitamin C family specifically called threonate, the body absorbs more of it. According to the same source, "the vitamin C threonate in Ester-C has been proven to reach white blood cells at levels nearly double the amount reached by other forms of vitamin C".

5.1. Ascorbic Acid vs. Ester-C

Ester-C is a patented form of Vitamin C (calcium ascorbate). Ester-C is non-acidic (pH neutral), which means it is more easily absorbed and is readily available to the body's cells in greater amounts than ascorbic acid. Its absorption is higher than ascorbic acid, and taken with full or low stomach. Also, Ester-C is retained in the body's cells for up to 24 hours which provides all-day protection. Ester-C contains natural flavonoids which are essential to boosting vitamin C's efficacy and its unique metabolite compounds make it more bioavailable in the body. Ester-C also supports white blood cells to fight infections. Also, it provides support during stress, cold and flu, and boosts vitamin C and calcium availability to bones and connective tissues. Ester-C is recommended for people with sensitive stomach lining like a peptic ulcer. It is recommended for a period of 3 to 6 months, both for adults and for children older than 12 years. Dosage form - tablets to be taken with a glass of water after meals.

Vitamin C, or ascorbic acid, is an essential antioxidant that is a powerful and effective ingredient in skin care products. Ascorbic acid is available in a number of forms, some of which are more efficacious than others. Ascorbic acid is a synthetic form of Vitamin C, derived from fermenting glucose, but the ascorbic acid molecule is not active in the body until it attaches to a mineral. Once bonded, the molecule works to neutralize free radicals, one of the root causes of skin aging, and reduces oxidative stress in the body. Vitamin C also increases the serum concentration of antioxidants, which helps to reverse DNA damage and neutralize free radicals. Vitamin C suppresses a pigment called melanin, protects the skin against sunburn, and increases collagen thickness, all of which aid in wrinkle reduction. The molecules of ascorbic acid are all straight. Generally, ascorbic acid is used in a tablet form.

6. Vitamin D

There are 2 primary forms of vitamin D—vitamin D2 (ergo-calciferol) and vitamin D3 (cholecalciferol). Vitamins D2 and D3 perform similar biological functions as a result of the hydration and dehydrogenation process. The primary difference between these two forms is their origin. Vitamin D2 is found in plants and fungi owing to ergosterol, while vitamin D3 is found in animal tissue owing to 7-DHC. Vitamin D3 is much more stable than D2 due to these plant and animal compounds. In one study, "rhythm M-values" were not significantly different in a cohort of Italian, non-diabetic obese individuals in metabolic syndrome, irrespective of the form of vitamin D administered. This aspect likely does not indicate a significant outcome and will not be included in any subsequent Vitamin D article.

It has been suggested that all the studies with no reported effect in vitamin D have been studies that used D2. As a result, D2 has been discarded by almost everyone and D3 has been favored in its place. However, there are still two primary forms of injectable vitamin D: Drisdol (D2) and Decara (D3). While vitamin D is best known for its impact on bone health, it also plays a substantial role in the immune system. The added benefit of subcutaneous and intramuscular vitamin D (as opposed to oral) is the potential contribution to mood regulation by preventing the development of chronic fatigue. Vitamin D in any form has been shown to reduce peripheral inflammation to increase the activity of T-cells. Vitamin D in either D2 or D3 forms accounts for the great majority of vitamin D deficiency cases, which is surprising in itself and well worth the extra discussion.

6.1. Vitamin D2 vs. Vitamin D3

However, when cholecalciferol and ergocalciferol are taken in similar amounts, they are considered similar. It is also important that the supplementation of dosages of up to 10,000 IU/day of both vitamin D2 or D3 is generally considered safe for adult consumption. On the other hand, animal studies have suggested that vitamin D2 increases inflammation rather than the ability of vitamin D3 to decrease inflammation. It has been shown that vitamin D3 increases circulating 25OHD concentration significantly more than vitamin D2 after a single large dose, indicating a lower bioavailability of D2. stated that the mean basal 25-hydroxyvitamin D concentrations after vitamin D2 administration were 4.88 ± 0.64 ng/mL, followed by those with regular doses of 2000 IU ranging from 15 to 19 ng/mL and 4000 IU with a range of 18.5–20 ng/mL. From their statement, it can be understood that vitamin D2 has a lower serum concentration as well as a worse impact on health. Furthermore, dosages of D2 ranging from 2000 IU and results in an average serum concentration of 15–20 ng/mL. In order to reach sufficient levels, the regular use of D2 would have to significantly lower dosages in milligrams and micrograms. D2 is also known as a provitamin because it has to be converted into a biologically active vitamin (metabolite) by the body and it does not immediately become a vitamin when it is processed by liver and kidney to get the necessary effect of vitamin D. With this being taken into account, D3 does not become a provitamin, does not need to be converted anymore, and is just used in the body directly. These differences are due to D3 being the most used and beneficial form of vitamin D than D2 because it is able to accomplish vitamin D's actual function. Thus, D2 is not the best type of vitamin D for the body and has poorer bioavailability.

Vitamin D has two natural forms— vitamin D2 (ergocalciferol) and vitamin D3 (cholecalciferol). The former form is produced from the ergosterol in mushrooms, whereas the latter form, previtamin D3, is produced from 7-dehydrocholesterol that is present in the skin of animals and humans. Both vitamin D3 and D2 are metabolized in the liver to 25-hydroxyvitamin D [25(OH)D] before being further converted to the biologically active form. According to some authors, the bioactivity of these compounds may differ. These differences are due to the limited bioavailability and different response in metabolic markers during hypocalciferolemic states. In recent years, cholecalciferol (vitamin D3) has been cited as the most beneficial form because cholecalciferol has been found to be more efficient than ergocalciferol at correcting vitamin D insufficiency and preventing deficiencies.

7. Vitamin E

Vitamin E helps to fight off free radicals in the body, allowing it to protect it from disease. There are two primary forms of vitamin E that our bodies use, and they have different abilities when it comes to absorption and bioavailability in the body. Vitamin E is fat-soluble in the body and, while it is absorbed in the small intestine, it is stored throughout all the tissues and organs in the body. In fact, over 93% of the vitamin E found in the body is stored in the fat tissues and muscle tissues from foods, but low levels are also found in the red blood cells. The two forms of vitamin E are alpha-tocopherol and tocotrienols. While alpha-tocopherol is the form most commonly used in supplements, this form of vitamin E received a scam rating with a low absorption and bioavailability of an estimated 11-39%. It is believed that this form of vitamin E is not very effective as it is not active.

Discovered in the mid-1920s, vitamin E is one of several naturally occurring fat-soluble antioxidants in the body. It plays a critical role in protecting your cells from oxidative damage. This is the kind of damage caused by free radicals that can build up and eventually lead to chronic diseases. Vitamin E was originally discovered because of its effect on fetal development. Research discovered that a dietary deficiency of vitamin E caused the fetus to reabsorb the placenta and die. Vitamin E has eight different forms: four types of tocopherols and four types of tocotrienols. The alpha-tocopherol form is best known for being involved in the birth process at preventing the fetus from dying, and studies have documented that low levels of alpha-tocopherol were associated with a risk of heart disease. More recent research has shown that the other forms of vitamin E, known as tocotrienols, may be even more powerful than alpha-tocopherol. In fact, a 2017 review investigated vitamin E tocotrienols for their absorption, metabolism, and potential health benefits in humans. It was noted that natural vitamin E tocotrienols, while being under-researched, had much better potential for health benefits compared to the synthetic form.

7.1. Alpha-Tocopherol vs. Tocotrienols

Discussion. The lipid-soluble compartment of cell plasma membranes consists of a non-polar or neutral layer sandwiched between another neutral layer. Free fatty acids, and to a lesser extent, cholesterol occupy the outer layer of the membrane facing the environment. The primary housekeeping lipid of the inner layer is phospholipids, with glycolipids and sphingolipids serving as minor components. Tocotrienols are not utilized outside of the cell due to rapid rates of metabolism and excretion (because they cannot be conserved with vitamin E transport proteins, VTPs). Non-polar molecules like T3s and T4s (and α-T) can move directly through the fatty acids of the outer layer and get into the membrane. In contrast, molecules like D-α- and D-δ-TMPs are polar because of the methyl substitution on the chromanol head, which allows electrons to delocalize in the benzene ring. These positively charged hydrogen atoms bind to the negatively charged phosphates of the inner layer unless the hydroxyl group is esterified to a phosphate; they don't contribute to plasma membrane resistance as does the phenol hydroxyl group.

Tocotrienols (T3) and tocopherols (T) are the two main forms of vitamin E, with the latter mostly cited as alpha-tocopherol (ATF/α-T). α-T has taken many of the accolades over the years, with its superior absorption and bioactivity in comparison to other T3s and T isomers; however, this is not completely substantiated. The allocated functional activities of these compound classes far outweigh differences in their absorption, but it is worth being aware of these when considering changes to the current evidence base related to specific health outcomes with T3 supplementation. For example, having supplements that have a known absorption profile could help in challenging individuals to take less frequent and higher doses of T3s for therapeutic outcomes, though these results would need to be better substantiated in the literature.

8. Vitamin K

Vitamin K is the fat-soluble nutrient responsible for blood clotting and bone metabolism. Dietary vitamins K1 and K2 are different components, but information on their ingestion, distribution, and metabolism is constantly growing and provides evidence that their effect as an essential nutrient should be documented. The majority of the vitamin K that the body needs comes from vegetables, especially leafy greens. You can get two kinds of vitamin K in your diet – vitamin K1, which is mainly found in green vegetables, and vitamin K2, which is mostly found in animal products. Once ingested, vitamin K1 can reduce platelet function, while vitamin K2 can activate the protein function that inhibits calcification.

Even though we have offered an ingredient or nutritional with a specific headline, we seldom prepare supplements with only one factor. Vitamins K1 and K2 are no different. Supplement K1 and K2 are the same in their verify/off breadth and also have a quick recommendation that is probably beneficial to those interested in optimum substances.

Can you worry about vitamin K? We think you should. Vitamin K is actually a very well-liked nutrient (most docs won't assess your vitamin K levels even though they review almost every other markers). Still, this vitamin is vital for your blood clotting components. That's why you should read this blog post about vitamins K1 and K2.

8.1. K1 vs. K2

It is important in bone formation and has demonstrated advantages on cardiovascular, cancer, bone health, immunomodulatory, and renal physiology. Studies show that it is often higher in its effectiveness against osteoporosis than K1. A small amount of K1 is converted to K2. Supplements of vitamin K1 and K2 may be taken by people with inadequate intake. Studies show that below 20% receptors promote K1 absorption while this increases to 80-90% receptors in the case of K2. Neither K1's absorption is affected by the presence or nature of a meal, nor are its absorption patterns over a short period of time reflective of vitamin K1 stored for use over an extended period of time, e.g. in your body or liver.

Vitamin K constitutes a group of chemicals; two important forms are K1 (phylloquinone) and K2 (menaquinone). K1 is primarily synthesized by plants and is present in green leafy vegetables and other plants. K2 is synthesized by animals and is present in dairy and meat products, with a few fermented food sources. K1 is predominantly responsible for clotting of blood, manufactured as well as obtained from plant food sources, and generally removed quickly from the blood by the liver after performing its clotting function. K2 has various subtypes, particularly MK4 and MK7, of which MK7 is biologically more effective.

9. Minerals and Their Absorption

Some of them have been mentioned below which are responsible for decreasing their absorption. 1) Oxalate and Phytate; both are naturally occurring compounds in fruit and vegetables. Both these compounds are responsible for inhibiting calcium absorption. Calcium oxalate and calcium phosphate are concerning factors when we look at kidney stone development. 2) Salt/Sodium; increases calcium excretion and decreases calcium absorption. A high-salt diet increases urinary calcium excretion. When the diet has calcium and sodium together, there is a decreased amount of calcium in the body through the urine process. 3) Protein; A high protein diet has increased the risk of mineral excretion which may lead to an increased calcium loss in the bone. The important point from the above factors is that iron, calcium, magnesium, potassium deficiency through food or supplements seem to be good, but due to poor solubility, it does not benefit greatly. Additionally, several other factors such as stress, aging, inflammation interfere with the absorption of minerals. It is an established fact that a small size particle of calcium magnesium citrate chelate and other minerals will be helpful in the absorption in the gastrointestinal tract.

Like vitamins, there are several types of minerals which a human body needs in trace and major quantities for better growth, development, and a healthy life. Minerals like calcium, iron, sodium, magnesium, potassium, phosphorus, and other minerals are essential for better body functioning. When we talk about minerals and their absorption, we need to understand that when these minerals are not soluble or absorbable properly by the body, they start storing in the body, building up in the body which brings several abnormalities and causes not only a single disease but a group of diseases. Out of these, the major minerals are calcium, magnesium, and iron which are considered problems of absorption.

9.1. Calcium

After calcium is consumed in food or supplements, it dissolves in the stomach and is then absorbed into the small intestine. At this point, foods and nutrients from other foods are absorbed at the same time, which may affect calcium absorption. Once absorbed, calcium moves into two places: bones and teeth, where it combines with phosphate to form the crystalline structure of the bones and teeth, and soft tissues. In the kidneys, calcium is filtered out of the blood and passes into the urine as a waste product.

Bone deposits are necessary to ensure strong bones. If not enough calcium is consumed in the diet, bone breakdown must replenish the body's calcium supply. Over time, the resulting bone loss can weaken the bones, making them fragile and causing the disease osteoporosis. Thus, sufficient dietary calcium is necessary to make sure that the bones are strong and healthy. Calcium intake from diet and supplements should not exceed 2,500 mg per day.

Calcium is a mineral crucial for bone health, muscle function, and nerve transmission. A steady supply of calcium is critical, as it is easily lost from the body. The average adult's body contains about 1.5-2 pounds (0.7-0.9 kg) of calcium. Ninety-nine percent of this is stored in the bones and teeth, while the remaining 1% is in the blood and other tissues. Although the calcium in your bones seems to function as a storage place for your body's calcium, it is much more than that. Bone undergoes continuous remodeling, with constant resorption and deposition of calcium into new bone.

10. Conclusion

The research reported in this paper was to get details of vitamins and minerals and their sources. They metallodrug compounds that should not be in touch with a food mechanism, while the vitamin dietary supplements should be similar to vitamins. The most efficient man-made vitamins and minerals, the types of minerals and vitamins, are natural mineral and vitamin complexes in the molecular level in the structure of the nanoemulsion. Study of drug delivery nanoemulsion. There are many ways in which vitamins and minerals could be produced to deal with the patients' digestive tract problems and numerous minerals and vitamins could be used to help patients. Knowledge of the types of man-made vitamin drug mechanisms could be useful in the drug-processing system for this paper. The authors provide a proposal to develop vitamins as nanoemulsions in the nonuse of natural and organic mineral complexes as chemical nanoparticles and antioxidants so that patients will feel more comfortable. In the pharmacological pharmacy sector, antioxidants and vitamins that inhibit the action of some medicine and chemotherapy could be utilized. When a medication is taken and the patient is unconsciously exposed to some form of vitamin inside a natural nanoemulsion, it could be utilized inside the onset to increase the security of administering the medication. For the growth of the pharmaceutical sector, man-made vitamins and medicines in chemotherapies could be employed effectively. Bioactivity or the body's ability to absorb vitamins or minerals is the ability to profit from the vitamins that a farmer has by meeting the standards of those with sensory clues. When the human body has more than enough vitamins inside, the advantage then enters the patient or on whom the work morally approaches. Little vitamins are absorbed into the human body for all vitamins, and no vitamins are made that are caused by exhaustion. It is not permitted to add vitamins from synthetic material as part of safety data, without any essential purpose to the extent not covered in this Directive.

In conclusion, minerals and vitamins are essential in maintaining normal health. This depends on several factors for which the bioavailability of nutrients is of unique interest. Minerals and vitamins are linked to many factors involved, such as production and absorption of minerals and vitamins, their chemical and molecular structure, the aging of the digestive system, or physiological conditions and methods of food processing. Vitamins and also natural and organic mineral complexes exhibited excellent absorption ability.

10.1. Summary of Key Points

Overall, the general principle when choosing a multivitamin or individual supplement is to look for the form of vitamin or mineral that is best absorbed in the body. Minerals are typically chelated or in a specific form (e.g., picolinate, citrate) in supplements because they are considered to be better absorbed. Not only does the best form of a nutrient ensure better absorption in the body, but these vitamins and minerals have the research to support their effectiveness. Different manufacturers prepare formulations in different ways so it is best to obtain advice from relevant clinicians before using them. Vitamins are essential for many bodily functions and if one is deficient they need to be corrected by taking the correct form, either in individual form or in a multivitamin.

It is important to choose the best forms of vitamins to ensure optimal absorption and bioavailability. Nutrient content and form can differ between individual supplement and food products, so it's important to consider not only the types of vitamins you are taking, but also the form in which they are provided. There are several factors that affect nutrient absorption. The presence of other nutrients can improve nutrient bioavailability, while certain food components can negatively affect nutrient absorption. Some medications and dietary practices can also have an impact on nutrient availability. Many factors can affect nutrient absorption when taking a supplement, such as dose and the form of the vitamin or mineral, including whether it is taken with or without food.

Factors Affecting Absorption of Vitamins

1. Introduction to Vitamin Absorption

1.1. Different Forms of Vitamins

1.2. Importance of Absorption

2. Factors Influencing Absorption

Factors influencing absorption: Many factors influence the absorption of vitamins. An individual's vitamin needs can vary greatly depending on age, sex, growth and development, medical history, and diet. Non-modifiable factors related to an individual are his age, sex, medical history while the other factors which are modifiable and if known will contribute to increasing absorption. These modifiable factors affect an individual's health and response to diet and nutrition. The age of the individual plays a vital factor in absorption as the changes in the anatomy and physiology of the gut in neonates and elderly have an extreme effect on the absorption. Gut function, including hygiene or lack thereof, physiology of nutrient handling, and gut protein and enzyme metabolism is influenced by the state of the gut, immune response, subject genetics and diet. Infection, drugs, and surgery are also of great importance because of the increased nutrient requirement and loss. The dietary factors include the type of food, the concentration of vitamins in food and the complete nutrient intake during a meal. All these factors should be taken into account while designing any nutraceutical product.

Introduction: The human body has requirements for very minimal amounts of vitamins and minerals. The absorption of vitamins is influenced by a multitude of factors. These factors have to be kept in mind while planning formulations to increase absorption by making products in delivery systems to increase bioavailability. These factors also play a crucial role in making the strategies to increase absorption and achieve targeted treatment in dietary supplement or therapeutic nutraceuticals field. The availability of options leads to using the symptoms as the first evidence of deficiency with the confirmation of testing.

2.1. Age

An adequate intake of all vitamins is associated with normal physiological processes, and different factors can interfere with that absorption. When considering human health, there is an obvious need for a balanced intake of vitamins, although its dietary reference values should take into account specific age-related needs. In particular, children and the elderly have opposite trends for their specific needs. Infants and adolescents, in fact, have a greater per-unit body weight need for vitamins than adults due to the higher energy requirements per unit of body weight. In any case, it is recommended to administer them supplements at the reference nutrient intake because these subjects have, on average, a reduced intake of food. Regarding the elderly, even though supplements can compensate for the lower energy intake, they are not absorbed, metabolized, or eliminated as effectively as in young people. Furthermore, the elderly have a higher individual response to drugs compared to adults, and using a potential variable drug response as the vitamin supplement would place them at risk for a suboptimal and unpredictable response. In conclusion, the high variability of the elderly in drug response and in age-related homeostenosis indicates that to optimize vitamin status and body function in the elderly, the nutrition community should also focus on the overall diet rather than on the use of the single vitamins.

Aging is associated with a number of physiological changes often referred to as homeostenosis that lead to decreased absorption of essential nutrients. Several factors might affect the nutritional status of subjects during their life course. On the one hand, there are changes that take place in the gastrointestinal tract and might interfere with an adequate absorption of nutrients, including vitamins and other micronutrients. On the other hand, older people consume a reduced quantity of food and sometimes they do not have access to nutrient-dense foods.

Niacin is stable in food and water. Milk, and to a lesser extent other foods, including meat, such as is on a pizza, yogurt, cottage cheese, and hard cheese, inhibit the absorption of niacin, while coffee and tea enhance it. In eastern and northern Europe, milk drinkers take in three times as much niacin due to coffee drinking and a greater than threefold increase in niacin compared with a modest intake of coffee or tea plus milk. Folic acid is found naturally in food and in the bread and flour that is fortified with folic acid in the U.S. B12 in food is bound to proteins and must be separated in the stomach for it to be absorbed. Animal proteins protect B12 and make it less available for absorption than purified B12. Pancreatic enzymes can then release B12 into an available form once proteins have been broken down. An acid environment is needed in the stomach for this process to work. B12 is commonly bound to plant proteins, which are not digested; hence, plant-source B12 is not absorbed.

Diet can often strongly influence absorption. There are various dietary substances that can enhance the absorption of different vitamins. Oranges and folic acid supplements will increase the absorption of iron, while high-calcium diets decrease it. Low-calcium diets may decrease zinc absorption. B vitamins are water soluble and should not be lost in traditional food preparation methods. It has been estimated that 50% of thiamin is lost in food preparation due to inappropriate cooking methods.

2.3. Gut Health

Gastric surgeries. In patients who undergo partial or total gastrectomy, protein absorption is usually somewhat decreased. Decreased motility of the small intestine can affect absorption as food is passed more slowly through the intestine so that the breakdown and absorption of nutrients are not perfect. Inflammation of the stomach or small or large intestine. This condition can occur in patients with chronic gastritis, chronic pancreatitis, acute or chronic hepatitis, etc. Decreased and thickening of the wall of blood capillaries. If the blood capillaries in the walls of the stomach, duodenum or village are disrupted by bleeding or thickened. Inflammation of the stomach. When experiencing an inflammatory condition in their stomach, a person will be difficult to absorb all kinds of vitamins, not only B group vitamins that play a role in the process of energy metabolism, but all other vitamins.

The condition of the gastrointestinal tract will have a major effect on the ability of the body to absorb nutrients. The innovative process of digestion and absorption occurs when the guts are in good shape. Therefore, it is very important to maintain good gut health by consuming nutrients from natural foods. If the condition of the body's internal organs is not good or has been disturbed, then we cannot expect nutrition to function properly in the body. In general, malabsorption of nutrients or absorption disorders can also occur due to various factors such as decreased gastric acid secretion. Decreased secretion of pepsin enzyme in the stomach so that protein is unable to break down into amino acids completely. Gluten intolerance, pancreatic insufficiency, impaired bile function, and dysfunctional intestines. The release of pancreatic juices is not optimal, so protein and fat cannot be broken down completely.

3. Techniques to Enhance Absorption

3. Certain vitamins and minerals require stomach acid to absorb. These include B-vitamins and such minerals as iron, calcium, magnesium, and zinc. Therefore, it's not recommended to take these supplements with antacids. That said, some sources say that the hydrochloric acid is the most important thing to consider, rather than the pH levels.

2. It is best to take vitamins with the food that has the... well, vitamins. For example, take a vitamin D supplement with a hobby that you might take outside like horseback riding, or take it with a meal of foods that are rich in vitamin D.

1. Take water-soluble vitamins with a meal. Vitamins like C, the B-vitamins, and folic acid can be taken on an empty or full stomach. Fat-soluble vitamins, however, are recommended to be taken with a meal and fat. They are more effectively absorbed when the concentration of fat in the intestines is highest, and that will happen after consuming a meal. Taking water-soluble vitamins with a meal might also be a good idea, especially for those with sensitive stomachs.

One of the most important elements of getting enough vitamins is spending the money on them and taking them consistently. In addition to doing that, the following techniques will help enhance absorption:

3.1. Combining Vitamins with Certain Foods

This is due to the inherent acidity of vitamin C and the antioxidizing effect of the compound that can counter magnesium. The avoidance of drinking coffee or tea 1 1/2 hours after meals might also help increase the iron uptake, as these drinks contain compounds that might bind to the minerals and prohibit their absorption. The toed condition can also accompany meals rich in fiber or could occur when calcium is consumed in high amounts, as this could interfere with the uptake of minerals. Examples of other food-vitamin interactions that potentially improve the bioavailability of vitamins are presented in other studies. For instance, a study on one fruit juice-vitamin C study found that consuming iron biofortified orange juice was 1.26- to 2.13-folds higher than drinking regular orange juice.

A strategy that can enhance the absorption of certain vitamins is to combine them with particular foods. By combining particular vitamins (from either food or supplements) with certain dietary factors, we can elicit the dietary activators of absorption and thereby improve the bioavailability of the studied vitamin. Vitamins that are fat-soluble, such as K, E, D, and A, are soluble in fat and should be combined with fat-containing foods. These fat-soluble vitamins should be mixed with unsaturated oils, such as vegetable and soy oils, as they enhance carotenoids or formulator, efficiently improving carotenoids absorption. These pairings have the potential to increase the bioavailability of vitamins, including vitamin C.

3.2. Taking Vitamins at Optimal Times

The right time to take a vitamin supplement can help increase bioavailability and boost the amount of vitamins or minerals that are actually absorbed by a person. Water-soluble vitamins dissolve in water, so they can be absorbed and utilized in the body quickly or excreted. Taking a water-soluble vitamin on an empty stomach can help boost absorption since an empty stomach means stomach juices or hydrochloric acid are not released to digest any ingested food - they will just be available in the stomach for absorbing the vitamin. A little bit of fat or a small meal can also help boost absorption of a fat-soluble vitamin. Fat-soluble vitamins - vitamins A, D, E, and K - are absorbed through the intestines with the help of fats. When the body is full of food, or in a fed state, it may slow the chemistry required to absorb or make use of the vitamin. This is why taking a vitamin supplement on an empty stomach may help boost absorption.

According to recent research, taking vitamins with food enhances bioavailability and boosts absorption, although the relationship is complex and relies heavily on the type of vitamins and minerals being ingested, as well as the individual's health. Vitamins are absorbed in the small intestine, with the help of transporters or binding proteins. A vitamin deficiency, an overabundance of vitamins, or some other aspect of an individual's health or physiology, such as their genetic makeup, can impact levels of transporters, binding proteins, or anti-nutrients produced to help the body absorb vitamins. Some foods can also affect transporters' or binding proteins' operation.

3.3. Using Supplements with Bioavailability Enhancers

The possibilities are smaller if the manufacturer unites the supplement with its enhancer with the natural additive present in the food. The use of salt ascorbate may be useful in these and other applications, as it is a multibiological compound and has several beneficial properties for some pathologies, stress, among others. It is important to emphasize that adjuvants used to increase the bioavailability of a certain nutrient must also be safe to be ingested, for example, some food additives like EDTA are not recommended for inflammatory smoothie containing iodine.

Supplements with main as well as adjuvant ingredients may be prepared by using enhancers of bioavailability. But it is particularly important in the case of therapeutic supplements, which the consumer needs to have an improvement, and that we know were bad (food, stress, etc.). These enhancers can act throughout the whole process of absorption, i.e. from when the supplement is ingested to when the controller (vitamin) is really absorbed by the body. Possessing these activities can be used together or even separately, producing what are called multiple supplements, compounds of vitamins, minerals, etc., separated from the bioavailability enhancers. This can be an alternative for consumers, which individually have a deficiency in the absorption of a given nutrient; they can choose the bioavailability enhancer according to the location of the nutrient they want to be absorbed.

3.3. Using Supplements Containing Bioavailability Enhancers

4. Conclusion and Recommendations

It is recommended that certain measures be taken to improve the absorption of recommended vitamins and nutrients. For instance, if one is taking multivitamins that contain iron, calcium, or egg protein, vitamin D should be taken at a different time. Similarly, multivitamins with iron, magnesium, and calcium should be taken at different times, as they can all interfere with each other's absorption. Antacids should also be taken separately from oral vitamins because they can prevent absorption, and iron supplements should be kept in a dry place. If pills get wet and begin to look different than usual, they should be thrown out. Overall, the goal in this area should be to maximize the concentrations and changes in micronutrient levels through improved oral administration.

In conclusion, it is clear that many factors can affect the efficacy of orally administered vitamins. Major factors, such as the site of absorption, are typically constant, and there is usually little that can be done to change them. However, people can take measures such as eating foods that contain optimal amounts of vitamins or taking supplements with vitamins that are highly bioavailable. Additionally, avoiding certain substances such as alcohol and using medications carefully can maximize vitamin absorption. By using the principles established in this research, people can improve overall health and ensure that their bodies have proper quantities of essential nutrients.

4.1. Summary of Key Points

Vitamin B12 can be malabsorbed by some people when it is attached to proteins in food. So, 1% will replace animal foods with B12 supplements and get a higher percentage usage. Folate follows more or less the same absorption pathways, which are also blocked when various things are missing or present in excess in the gut. So, folic absorption can be negatively affected by lack of intrinsic factor and high serum gastrin. This means that we don't get much of a look-in about the influence of several other factors that govern B12 absorption because the majority of the population are not that dysfunctional for B12 absorption.

Taking Stock Both B12 and B9 have complex absorption pathways. Several different chemicals can close down different pathways to a greater or lesser extent, and some other compounds can make any closed pathways less of a problem. However, obviously, some combinations are particularly bad. The proof of the pudding in these cases is that taking mega-dose versions of the vitamins to swamp out the competitive or blocking compounds can bypass the absorption problem and restore serum levels and health. And, of course, if there is widespread malnutrition among a population, all of the non-absorptive pathways can get overwhelmed.

4.2. Practical Tips for Maximizing Vitamin Absorption

There are a few factors present in some food or food processing operations that limit the bioavailability of individual vitamins, such as the presence of inhibitors and poor matrix compatibility (that is not enough release from the food matrix) that limit the efficiency of absorption. Therefore, practical dietary advice on how to best maximize the absorption of vitamins may result in a better intake and better status of these micronutrients. The following are tips and tricks for improving the absorption of vitamins.

In addition to the discussed concepts and principles, some practical tips are provided for maximizing the absorption of vitamins. A few factors that have been shown to improve nutrient utilization in general are probiotics/prebiotics, bile salts, and fermentation by-products such as short-chain fatty acids. Of interest, some of the discussed vitamins, like vitamin E, A, and K, have demonstrated to have positive effects on gut health. Therefore, future research could benefit from investigating the effects on gut health not only of vitamins but also of other food bioactives or plant compounds in innovative food matrices. Indeed, there are many conditions and dietary habits that impair the efficient utilization of vitamins and minerals, particularly in the elderly population. There are also circumstances where people suffer from vitamin deficiencies regardless of their dietary intake and neither oral vitamin nor mineral supplements, nor fortified products, can raise the status of proportion of people. Thus, specific dietary guidelines capable of providing the maximum amount of these nutrients under diverse circumstances are essential.

www.ingramcontent.com/pod-product-compliance
Lightning Source LLC
Chambersburg PA
CBHW071108260726
48661CB00006B/2530